THE STRESS OVERCOMING TIPS.

How to free your mind from stress.

BY

Marthins Kelly

Copyright©2023

TABLE OF CONTENTS

Chapter 1: INTRODUCTION

Chapter 2: HOW STRESS AFFECTS YOUR MENTAL HEALTH.

Chapter 3: STRESS COMES IN MANY FORMS.

Chapter 4: EXERCISE CAN RELIEVE STRESS.

Chapter 5: USING MUSIC THERAPY FOR STRESS RELIEf.

Chapter 6: STRESS RELIEF VACATIONS.

Chapter 7: HEALTHY BODY AND MIND FOR STRESS RELIEF.

Chapter 8: GETTING RID OF STRESS WITHOUT DRUGS.

Chapter 9: USING ART THERAPY FOR STRESS RELIEF.

Chapter 10: STRESS RELIEF FOR MEN AND WOMEN.

Chapter 1:

INTRODUCTION

Stress can affect anyone at any time, and it can be caused by various factors such as work, relationships, or health issues. Overcoming stress requires a multifaceted approach that involves lifestyle changes, stress management techniques, and seeking professional help if necessary.

Stress is a common experience that everyone goes through at some point in their lives. It is the body's natural response to a challenge or demand. While some stress can be beneficial and motivate individuals to take action, too much stress can have negative effects on both physical and mental health.

When an individual experiences stress, the body releases hormones such as cortisol and adrenaline. These hormones prepare the body for a fight or flight response, which can cause physical symptoms such as increased heart rate, rapid breathing, and tense muscles.

In the short term, stress can be helpful in improving performance and increasing focus. However, chronic stress can lead to a range of health problems such as high blood pressure, heart disease, and mental health issues like anxiety and depression.

Managing stress is important for overall health and wellbeing. Some effective ways to manage stress include practicing mindfulness, exercise, getting enough sleep, and engaging in activities that bring joy and relaxation. Seeking support from friends, family, or a mental health professional can also be helpful in managing stress.

If you are experiencing chronic stress or feel overwhelmed, it's important to seek help from a healthcare provider or mental health professional. They can provide guidance and support to help you manage your stress and improve your overall wellbeing.

Chapter 2:

HOW STRESS AFFECTS YOUR MENTAL HEALTH.

Stress can have a significant impact on your health. Some common physical symptoms of stress include headaches, muscle tension, fatigue, and difficulty sleeping. Long-term stress can also weaken the immune system and increase the risk of developing chronic health conditions such as heart disease, diabetes, and depression. It's important to manage stress through healthy coping mechanisms such as exercise, meditation, and spending time with loved ones.

Anxiety disorder is a mental health condition that can cause feelings of worry, fear, and apprehension. Some common symptoms of anxiety disorder include excessive worry, restlessness, fatigue, trouble concentrating, irritability, muscle tension, and sleep disturbances. Treatment for anxiety disorder typically involves a combination of therapy and medication. Cognitive-behavioral therapy (CBT) and exposure therapy are common forms of therapy used to treat anxiety disorder. Anti-anxiety medications, such as benzodiazepines and beta-blockers, may also be prescribed by a doctor to help manage symptoms. It's important to seek professional help if you believe you may be experiencing symptoms of anxiety disorder.

Chapter 3:

STRESS COMES IN MANY FORMS.

Stress is a common experience that can affect people in many different ways. It can come in many forms, from physical stress like chronic pain or illness, to mental and emotional stress like anxiety or depression. Work-related stress, financial stress, and relationship stress are also some of the most common stressors people experience.

In addition, stress can be acute or chronic, meaning it can be a short-term or long-term experience. Acute stress is usually caused by a specific event, like a deadline or a sudden change in plans, while chronic stress is more ongoing and can be caused by a variety of factors.

It's important to recognize when you are experiencing stress and to take steps to manage it. This can include things like exercise, meditation, therapy, or simply taking time for yourself to relax and recharge. By recognizing and managing stress, you can help prevent long-term health problems and improve your overall well-being.

Anxiety symptoms relief disorder can be a challenging condition to manage, especially when traditional treatments are not effective. However, there are still options available for those struggling with anxiety. Here are some possible ways to manage anxiety symptoms when traditional treatments are not working:

Psychotherapy: Also known as talk therapy or psychological counseling, psychotherapy involves working with a therapist to reduce your anxiety symptoms. It can be an effective way to manage anxiety symptoms when traditional treatments are not working.

Medication: While medication cannot cure anxiety disorder, it can improve symptoms and help you function better. Medications for anxiety disorders often include antidepressants, anti-anxiety medications, and beta-blockers.

Alternative treatments: There are various alternative treatments for anxiety disorder, including mindfulness, relaxation techniques, correct breathing techniques, dietary adjustments, and more.

Support from loved ones: Having a support system can be extremely helpful for those struggling with anxiety disorder. Friends and family members can provide emotional support and help with practical tasks.

Combination therapy: For some individuals, a combination of psychotherapy, medication, and/or alternative treatments may be the most effective way to manage anxiety symptoms. It's important to work with a healthcare professional to determine the best treatment plan for your unique situation.

Stress is a natural response to the challenges and demands of daily life. While some stress is necessary for motivation and optimal performance, excessive or chronic stress can have negative effects on both physical and mental health.

The effects of stress can manifest in different ways. Some common physical symptoms of stress include headaches, muscle tension, fatigue, and sleep disturbances. Mentally, stress can lead to anxiety, irritability, and difficulty concentrating. Prolonged stress can also increase the risk of developing chronic health conditions such as cardiovascular disease, diabetes, and depression.

Fortunately, there are many remedies for managing stress. One effective way to reduce stress is through relaxation techniques such as deep breathing, meditation, or yoga. Exercise is also a great way to reduce stress and improve overall health. Maintaining a healthy diet, getting enough sleep, and practicing good time-management skills can also help to reduce stress levels.

Another important remedy for stress is social support. Talking to friends or family members about your stress can help you to gain perspective and feel less isolated. Professional counseling or therapy can also be helpful for those experiencing chronic or severe stress.

In summary, while stress is a natural part of life, it is important to manage it effectively in order to maintain physical and mental health. By practicing relaxation techniques, maintaining a healthy lifestyle, and seeking social support when needed, individuals can reduce the negative effects of stress and improve their overall well-being.

Chapter 4:

EXERCISE CAN RELIEVE STRESS.

Exercise is a great way to relieve stress. When we exercise, our bodies release endorphins, which are natural mood-boosters that help to reduce stress and anxiety. Additionally, exercise can help distract us from our worries and problems, giving us a mental break and helping us to feel more relaxed.

There are many different types of exercise that can be great for stress relief. Cardiovascular exercises, such as running or biking, can be especially effective for releasing endorphins and reducing stress. Yoga and other types of stretching can also be great for stress relief, as they can help to loosen tight muscles and promote relaxation.

It's important to note that while exercise can be a great tool for stress relief, it's not a cure-all. If you're experiencing chronic stress or anxiety, it's important to seek professional help from a mental health care provider. Nonetheless, incorporating regular exercise into your routine can help to reduce stress and improve your overall well-being.

Exercise and stress relief have a very healthy relationship. Regular exercise can be an excellent way to relieve stress and improve your overall mental health. When you exercise, your body releases endorphins, which are natural chemicals that can help to reduce stress and promote feelings of happiness and well-being. Additionally, exercise can help to clear your mind and provide a healthy outlet for negative emotions and stress.

Incorporating exercise into your daily routine can be an effective way to manage stress. This could include activities such as running, walking, cycling, swimming, or practicing yoga. Even just a few minutes of exercise each day can make a big difference in your stress levels and overall mental health.

It's important to remember that exercise should be used as a tool to manage stress, not as a way to escape from it. It's also important to consult with your healthcare provider before starting any new exercise routine. With consistency and commitment, you can build a healthy relationship between exercise and stress relief that will benefit your physical and mental well-being.

Chapter 5:

USING MUSIC THERAPY FOR STRESS RELIEf.

Music therapy is a form of therapy that uses music to promote emotional, physical, and mental well-being. It has been found to be effective in reducing stress and anxiety, and promoting relaxation.

Listening to music can help to slow down breathing and heart rate, which can help to reduce feelings of stress and anxiety. It can also help to distract your mind from negative thoughts and feelings, and help you to focus on the present moment.

Music therapy can be personalized to the individual's needs, preferences, and goals. A trained music therapist can use a variety of techniques, such as playing instruments, singing, and improvisation, to help clients achieve their therapeutic goals.

In addition to reducing stress and anxiety, music therapy has been found to be effective in treating depression, improving communication and social skills, and promoting physical rehabilitation. It is a safe and non-invasive form of therapy that can be used in conjunction with other treatments.

Overall, music therapy is a powerful tool for stress relief and can be used by anyone, regardless of musical ability or background. So, the next time you are feeling stressed or anxious, try putting on some calming music and see how it can positively impact your mood.

Chapter 6:

STRESS RELIEF VACATIONS.

Stress relief vacations have become increasingly popular in recent years, as more people look for ways to relax and recharge from their busy lives. These vacations are designed to help people reduce their stress levels and improve their overall well-being.

There are many different types of stress relief vacations available, depending on your interests and preferences. Some popular options include yoga retreats, meditation retreats, spa vacations, and nature retreats. Many of these vacations offer a combination of activities, such as yoga and meditation classes, spa treatments, hiking, and healthy meals.

One of the benefits of stress relief vacations is that they can help you disconnect from technology and daily stressors. By immersing yourself in a peaceful environment and focusing on relaxation and self-care, you can reduce your stress levels and improve your mental and physical health.

If you're interested in taking a stress relief vacation, there are many resources available to help you plan your trip. You can research different options online, read reviews from other travelers, and consult with a travel agent or wellness specialist to find the perfect vacation for you. Remember, taking care of your mental and physical health is important, and a stress relief vacation can be a great way to prioritize self-care and relaxation.

Stress relief vacations can be a great way to unwind and recharge your batteries. There are many places around the world that offer peaceful environments, beautiful scenery, and relaxation activities that can help you forget about the daily grind. Here are a few places that are great for stress relief vacations:

1. Bali, Indonesia - Bali is known for its beautiful beaches, lush jungles, and tranquil temples. You can spend your days practicing yoga, getting massages, and soaking in natural hot springs.

2. Sedona, Arizona - Sedona is a desert oasis that offers stunning red rock formations, hiking trails, and spiritual retreats. You can join a guided meditation session, explore the local art galleries, or take a hot air balloon ride.

3. Tulum, Mexico - Tulum is a beautiful coastal town that offers white sandy beaches, turquoise waters, and Mayan ruins. You can spend your days practicing yoga on the beach, snorkeling in the coral reefs, or exploring the local markets.

4. Banff, Canada - Banff is a picturesque mountain town that offers stunning views of snow-capped peaks, crystal clear lakes, and hiking trails. You can spend your days skiing, snowshoeing, or relaxing in natural hot springs.

5. Kyoto, Japan - Kyoto is a beautiful city that offers traditional Japanese gardens, temples, and cultural experiences. You can spend your days practicing meditation, learning calligraphy, or exploring the local tea houses.

Chapter 7:

HEALTHY BODY AND MIND FOR STRESS RELIEF.

Maintaining a healthy body and mind is crucial for stress relief. Here are some tips you can follow to achieve this:

1. Exercise regularly: Exercise can help reduce stress and anxiety by releasing endorphins, which are natural mood-boosters. Aim for at least 30 minutes of moderate exercise, such as jogging or cycling, most days of the week.

2. Get enough sleep: Lack of sleep can increase stress levels and impact your mood. Aim for 7-8 hours of sleep each night to help promote a healthy mind and body.

3. Eat a healthy diet: Eating a balanced diet rich in fruits, vegetables, whole grains, and lean protein can help fuel your body and mind, and reduce stress.

4. Practice relaxation techniques: Techniques such as deep breathing, meditation, and yoga can help reduce stress and promote relaxation.

5. Stay connected: Social support can help reduce stress and boost mood. Stay connected with friends and family through phone calls, video chats, or social media.

Remember, maintaining a healthy body and mind takes time and effort, but the benefits are worth it.

Chapter 8:

GETTING RID OF STRESS WITHOUT DRUGS.

Stress is a common problem that affects many people. While there are drugs that can help alleviate stress, there are also many ways to reduce stress without drugs. Here are a few ways you can get rid of stress without taking medication:

1. Exercise: Regular exercise is a great way to reduce stress. Exercise releases endorphins, which are natural mood enhancers. It also helps to reduce tension in the body, which can help to reduce stress.

2. Meditation: Meditation is a great way to reduce stress. It helps to calm the mind and reduce anxiety. There are many different types of meditation, so finding one that works for you is important.

3. Deep breathing: Deep breathing is a simple technique that can help to reduce stress. Take slow, deep breaths in through your nose and out through your mouth. This helps to slow down your heart rate and reduce tension.

4. Get enough sleep: Lack of sleep can increase stress levels. Make sure you get enough sleep each night to help reduce stress.

5. Eat a healthy diet: Eating a healthy diet can help to reduce stress. Make sure you eat plenty of fruits, vegetables, and whole grains, as well as lean protein sources.

Chapter 9:

USING ART THERAPY FOR STRESS RELIEF.

Art therapy is a great way to relieve stress and improve mental health. Through the use of various art forms such as painting, drawing, and sculpting, individuals can express themselves and explore their emotions in a safe and creative way.

Research has shown that art therapy can help reduce symptoms of anxiety, depression, and post-traumatic stress disorder. It can also improve self-esteem and help individuals better understand their thoughts and feelings.

One of the benefits of art therapy is that it does not require any artistic talent or skill. The focus is on the process of creating rather than the final product. This allows individuals to let go of any self-judgment or expectations and simply enjoy the act of creating.

Art therapy can be done individually or in a group setting, and it is often used in conjunction with other types of therapy. It is important to note that art therapy should not be used as a substitute for professional treatment, but rather as a complementary tool.

If you are interested in trying art therapy for stress relief, there are many resources available. You can look for a licensed art therapist in your area or try online resources such as virtual art therapy sessions or guided art activities. Remember, the goal of art therapy is not to create a masterpiece, but rather to use art as a tool for self-expression and stress relief.

Chapter 10:

STRESS RELIEF FOR MEN AND WOMEN.

1. Exercise regularly: Exercise is a great way to relieve stress. It releases endorphins, which are natural mood boosters, and helps to reduce stress hormones like cortisol.

2. Practice relaxation techniques: Relaxation techniques like deep breathing, meditation, and yoga can help to calm your mind and reduce stress levels.

3. Write it down: Writing down your thoughts and feelings can help to release tension and reduce stress.

4. Talk to someone: Talking to a friend or family member can help to relieve stress and provide emotional support.

5. Get organized: Being organized can help to reduce stress levels by providing a sense of control and reducing clutter.

6. Focus on what you can control: Instead of worrying about things you cannot control, focus on the things you can control, and take action.

7. Embrace the mess: Accept that life can be messy, and don't try to control every aspect of it.

Remember, managing stress is different for everyone. Finding what works for you is key to reducing stress and improving your mental health.

www.ingramcontent.com/pod-product-compliance
Lightning Source LLC
Chambersburg PA
CBHW031600210526
45464CB00003B/1371